Calisthenics Training

3 weeks Bodyweight Program to get Fast Fat
Burning and Strength results
Copyright © 2020
All rights reserved.

ISBN

Disclaimer

The information contained in *Calisthenics training* " is

meant to serve as a comprehensive collection of strategies that the author of this eBook has done research about. Summaries, strategies, tips and tricks are only recommendation by the author, and reading this eBook will not guarantee that one's results will exactly mirror the author's results. The author of the eBook has made all reasonable effort to provide current and accurate information for the readers of the eBook. The author and it's associates will not be held liable for any unintentional error or omissions that may be found. The material in the eBook may include information by third parties. Third party materials comprise of opinions expressed by their owners. As such, the author of the eBook does not assume responsibility or liability for any third party material or opinions. Whether because of the progression of the internet, or the unforeseen changes in company policy and editorial submission guidelines, what is stated as fact at the time of this writing may become autdated or inapplicable later.

The eBook is copyright © 2020 with all rights reserved. It is illegal to redistribute , copy, or create derivative work from this eBook whole or in part. No parts of this report may be reproduced or retransmitted in any reproduced or retransmitted in any forms whatsoever without the writing expressed and signed permission from the author.

Contents

WHAT EXACTLY IS CALISTHENICS TRAINING?

Calisthenics is quickly becoming one of the most sought after pieces of training that gymnasts, coaches, and trainers incorporate into their fitness programs to further improve the efficiency of their workouts.

What Exactly Is Gymnastics?

In short, these are in fact exercises that include only body weight. It may include the use of equipment but is not necessary. These exercises include, but are not limited to, jumps, handles, swinging, chin, etc. All of these exercises increase flexibility, muscle coordination, and mobility.

There are many examples of Calisthenics training that you can include in your workout. In this Book, we will focus on three important muscle groups, namely the chest, back, and legs.

For chest muscles, the most common exercise is push-ups. There are many variations of the handle that can be made, namely flat, oblique and rejected. Standard push-ups include one that holds the arms and legs apart in the shoulder width. When performing push-up exercises, the back should be kept in a neutral position to avoid unnecessary strain on the spine.

 If this exercise is too difficult, especially for someone who has not trained for a long time, it may be good to lay your knees on the ground. This facilitates exercise. Angled and rejected handles can be made using easily accessible objects such as seats or stairs etc.

For the rear muscles, the most common exercise is the chin or thrust, which is known in the fitness literature. Some consider chin one of the most difficult functions.

There are also various variations, such as the upper and lower handles, or in terms of separating the width of both hands. If you are unable to perform at least one chin, first try a passive and active pause for at least 15-20 seconds and try at least 5 negative moves. This builds your base in the back muscles and helps you move to your first chin.

Finally, there are many gymnastic exercises for the leg muscles that train different parts of the legs. Let's look at the most common one that is a squat. It trains your quadriceps muscle and is extremely easy. Just go back and forth so that your knees are not over your toes. This avoids unnecessary strain on the knees.

That is all! These are 3 simple weight gain exercises that you can use to effectively train your chest, back, and legs. There are many other exercises in gymnastics that you can integrate into your workout plan.

You can even combine with resistance training to further improve the performance of your training program.

Benefits of Calisthenics for a quick training
Calisthenics - Benefits of explaining speed explained

Calisthenics is ideal for getting fit and running the neck speed you need to get trophies and headlines. However, some runners and quick training athletes think that gymnastics is not necessary to speed up. And some have the misconception that training in gymnastics slows you down. It cannot be further from the truth. The following gymnastic benefits for speed training should solve this matter nicely.

Features variations in your workout

One of the best benefits of gymnastics training is that you have many variations in your speed training. When integrating knee heights, handles, crunches and plates with very little rest between sets, you assume that your body is as fast as possible. Be sure to keep pushing and try different exercises to make your body even more conditioned.

Improves coordination

When you talk about the benefits of gymnastics for speed training, you can't lose sight of coordination. Coordination plays a big role in how fast you are and when your coordination is a little off, you can't increase sales and other runners will eventually blow you up. But if you train different gymnastics several times a week, you will be much better coordinated and as a result, your speed will increase.

You get stronger

One of the most obvious advantages of gymnastics in speed training is the fact that you are strengthening with each session. Of course, you need to make sure that you have enough fuel when it comes to healthy food and drink and that you have enough rest, but if you do gymnastics in the form of pushups and braces and all the exercises you normally do during exercise, stronger and increases your strength and your speed.

Hopefully, you are convinced that you need calisthenics in your training plan if you want to develop a speed that others, including scouts, will notice. You don't want to be the slowest person in the field and you don't want to be second. You want to win, so you train every opportunity you get with all the tools you have learned to bring you to your winning goals.

But if you don't add gymnastics with the rest of the tools, you will eventually reach your glass ceiling and stay there. Instead, realize the benefits of gymnastics for speed training and training as experts do. Calisthenics is not an "old school" or obsolete and will certainly not slow you down. Instead, they make you more coordinated, stronger and faster than ever. If you don't believe it, try including gymnastics in your routine and you will be guaranteed all the speed goals you achieve for yourself.

Calisthenic Training - The key to successful training

There are a thousand workouts, pills and diets that should help you with your health and fitness. Some of them help and inspire people, but others will trick you into short-term results that do not lead to the best health and fitness in the long run.

Keep in mind that when it comes to calisthenics, the winning approach must include your motivation, your training, and your diet.I will give you an overview of these three keys to achieving your health and health goals in the long run.Let's start with motivation. With motivation, we can look at your philosophy, your attitude, and your goals. Of course, objectives are very important.

You must first set a goal to reach the goal. The benefits of Calisthenic bodyweight workouts are so obvious that it seems impossible to forget them, and yet occasionally they do. We leave things in our way. We will let the other priorities catch up with our health and fitness. Yet our health and fitness is an area of our lives that has a positive impact on all other Aryans.

When setting your goals, you must touch several important reasons to have those goals. For example, I lose ten pounds, so I feel good about myself or walk two miles to keep up with my children and be a good parent. Set your goals, but be sure to give some strong reasons for achieving these goals. This is the only way to maintain high motivation in everyday life.

You must also look at your attitude and philosophy with motivation.

Attitude is a precursor to what you do. If you don't have good access, you probably don't have good actions. For example, if you think you don't have time for your calisthenics training, you are wrong. You have the wrong attitude and your priorities are confused. Before you ever want to change, you have to change your attitude.

If you don't do the right things and get the right results, take a look at what you think. Here you have control over your thoughts, not the other way around. You have to take control and your philosophy will help you with that.

Philosophy brings the attitude to a deeper level. You can choose your philosophy and choose what you accept. For example, in my life, I have a philosophy that calisthenics training is a must for duty and joy.

You need to look at your philosophy, attitude, and goals as you approach your health and fitness goals.Another important key is training. The best calisthenics exercises include three aspects: resistance weight training, cardiovascular weight training and flexibility training.

Calisthenic resistance training involves weight gain and is important for maintaining and increasing muscle tone and strength.Cardiovascular calisthenics exercises include fitness and weight gain and are great for burning body fat.Flexible training protects you from injury. It will help you maintain good posture and movement in all your seams.

Nutrition is the third important key. There is so much information that you do not know what to accept. However, you do not want to go on a diet, which is a short-term solution. You will learn about nutrition and learn the right principles of healthy eating.

When I was just starting to train for weight gain, I thought I should only do push-ups, squirts, and squats for bodybuilding. So I did them, I got good at those workouts and then hit the rig.

I completed many free weight programs and most of them were relatively similar. I needed something new and something more complete.

It is very important to distinguish between all different types of body weight, as any method can be used for a particular purpose. Basic physical exercises such as pushups, pullups, and bodyweight squats can be used for overall strength and fitness.

Calisthenic training, on the other hand, is more of a cardio exercise.

Because I age cardio at a steady state, I usually use body weight and other training methods to replace the need for cardio. But besides my aversion to steady-state cardio, there are other very important benefits of using very intense gymnastic training as a form of cardio:

One of the main benefits of Calisthenics is improved cardiorespiratory endurance, which is the ability of your body to capture, process, release and retain oxygen to create the energy needed to perform a certain activity completely.

It is characterized by a healthy and effective heart and lungs. Cardiorespiratory (cardio) stamina is probably more important than fat loss or muscle growth but is one of the least discussed aspects of fitness.

If you have more endurance in cardio, you can easily do more for longer. This will improve your ability to perform sports, work and life activities. If you combine basic gymnastics with weight training, you can train muscles and train the hearts and lungs.

This will help you perform other physical activities better. Most people are excited and exhausted while trying to perform simple tasks like lifting boxes on the stairs or trying to catch a bus.

These activities require physical fitness and fitness testing. Many rats in the gym are often injured because they quickly get tired. When your body is tired of strenuous exercise, it is a sign of poor healing.

Your muscles are not getting the right amount of oxygen for complete recovery. Fatigue leads to poor form, which in turn leads to personal injury. Generally, you will be much healthier if your heart and lungs become healthier.

With conditioning, you can essentially improve your ability to live life to the fullest. On the other hand, many brainwashed people are convinced that there is a specific "target heart zone" that will effectively help you burn fat and improve heart endurance.

This is false and such a zone does not exist. Athletes with the best cardiac endurance - the balance between a healthy heart and lung function and good physical fitness - are those who perform intense exercises such as sprinters.

In short, it can hardly last longer. Note, however, that exercise for physical gymnastics is very intense and difficult. You need to develop constantly, especially if you spent most of your time after cardio exercise published in most magazines.

Calisthenics exercise example

Lomax coach handles a large number of movements in gymnastics. Some of them you have heard about and may have even appeared before. But many of you will be brand new.

Here is a list of calisthenic movements that the trainer Lomax will teach you:

- Split jump
- Jumping jacks
- Simulated skipping rope
- Standing twist
- Well and bend
- windmill
- High knees
- Jogging on the spot

- marching

Calisthenic movements seem simple to you, but the key is to do them in advance. You can start by taking each exercise for 60 seconds and then immediately proceed to the next move.This circuit-style workout will be much more fun and exciting than a traditional type of cardio workout.

Once you are good at these basic calisthenic movements, you can begin with the Animal Calisthenics movement, which places more emphasis on the heart, lungs, and muscles.

6 main reasons why weight training is important

Do you need an expensive gym and access to all shiny machines or expensive equipment and magic powders to improve strength, fitness, and fitness?

Weight training is one of the most versatile, cost-effective and cost-effective training methods available to both serious athletes and non-professional fitness enthusiasts.

1. Calisthenics of body weight can be done anywhere

You don't need an expensive gym membership or

expensive equipment to benefit from physical gymnastics ... you have everything you need now and now.

Inside or outside ... there are several exercises for weight training that you can perform to greatly improve strength, fitness, and fitness.

2. Calisthenics for body weight is an ideal place to start

If you're just starting with a fitness training program .weight training is an ideal place to start.Gymnastics prepares you with a physical foundation from which you can effectively and safely add advanced resistance training.

Learn how to control your body weight before exploring other training methods.

3. Bodyweight gymnastics can be adjusted for each level of fitness.There are many variations to workout in a gym with weight ... so you can make it easier or more difficult.

Therefore, they are good for both beginners and experienced fitness enthusiasts.

4. Calisthenics of bodyweight Exercise natural body movement.Resistance training methods often do not directly improve the movement patterns that are

naturally used in everyday life ... but this is not the case with bodyweight gymnastics.

Fitness perfection is often measured by your ability to control the movements of your body ... and not by your ability to control the movement of an object.

Train as you move naturally to see more physical enhancements that relate to the real world.

5. Gymnastics with body weight can improve muscle strength, strength, and endurance

Depending on the exercises used, reps and sets and intensity ... you can access strength, strength, and endurance individually or together.

The challenges of sport, work, and life rarely differ in one-dimensional ... but rather in a combination of strength, strength, and endurance.

The gym is a great way to train all three and flow smoothly from one power to another.

6. Gymnastics with body weight can simultaneously improve strength and cardiovascular endurance in fat burning.When most of us participate in a fitness

training program, we want to improve strength and cardiovascular endurance ... while burning unwanted fat.

Gymnastics can do all three ... in the same exercise.

By changing exercise, stress, and training intensity, you can effectively and effectively become stronger, better conditioned and leaner

Do not be fooled by the simplicity of gymnastics with bodyweight ... are one of the best tools you have for increasing strength, fitness, and fitness.

And because it looks simple, it doesn't mean they're light or ineffective ... try a one-arm push-up, one-arm pull-up with one leg if you don't believe me.

Weight training should be the foundation of any physical training program ... It is the ideal place to start and should remain an important part of your fitness training program as you add more workouts.

HOW TO SLIM DOWN, AGILE, STRONG, MUSCULAR AND HEALTHY

Weight loss is not as difficult as you think. Weight loss or slimming down is not difficult at all, even if you are very, very fat. slimming down can only be achieved in eight simple steps. These steps can be taken by anyone, be it a child or an adult, old or young, woman or man. Weight loss, as described in these steps, does not require going to the gym, not exercising vigorously and not spending money. If you follow this simple weight loss guide, you can lose weight after approximately two weeks. This diet guide has been prepared with great attention. If you read it, you will understand that it is not written with a specific business motif. It is written in layman language so you can easily follow it. It is designed to help you and people like you who are concerned about weight loss, who spend their valuable money on consulting dietitians and doctors and visiting gyms who believe that weight loss can only be achieved through extensive and exhaustive training. by driving twenty kilometers every day by cutting tasty meals, tasty meals, sweets, and chocolate.

Part 1: Slimming Myths

Stop feeling guilty for jumping: you have not broken any law

First of all, remember that if you are obese, fat, obese and look ugly, you should never feel guilty. Eating is one of the best hobbies you can have. Those who laugh at your bloated figure are cruel, naughty and foolish. Remember that those who are slim and thin are almost always bad because they constantly miss out on one of the greatest joys of their lives. You should never feel guilty about being fat, you should never collect yourself for it. You like food. It is not a crime. The first criterion for diets is that you are free from guilt and that you must be brave enough to tell yourself that you have done nothing wrong by eating your favorite food. I do not know how many dietitians you have visited or how many doctors you have seen, but I am sure none of them have told you that "eating is an extremely enjoyable pastime and that you feel guilty because you are food." "

You will lose weight. Do you not want to die?

Yes, doctors and dietitians are like that. They tend to

scare you. Some may have prescribed diet pills. I hope you didn't take one. Never take pills to be on a diet, regardless of who prescribed them. They cause cancer.

Many people take into account that medication helps them to lose weight easily without having to reduce their diet or the intake of high-fat foods. They think that slimming tablets make them thin like a tear while they continue to enjoy chocolate, spaghetti, ice cream, and other bans and junk foods. The diet pills undoubtedly make them thin, but within a few years, they do not know whether they have become thin because of the pills or because of cancer caused by the pills in their body.

Exercise is not bad

Another point that doctors and dietitians continue to play drums is sports. Now understand this carefully: Exercise beyond a certain level is for your health. If you think that by spending hours and money in the gym you get the enviable number you want, think again. Spending so many hours at the gym is difficult to lose or not to lose, but you certainly get a heart attack. Accurate, rigorous and energetic workouts damage the heart. Some of the best and thinnest actors in the world are heart patients, precisely because of too much training in the gym.

Training sensible and normal

It is not necessary for you to destroy your sleep of beauty, to get up in the early hours of the morning and run around the neighborhood or run around a monument or do yoga. Sleep is very important to the body. So please sleep well. Get up when the time comes, otherwise, you'll be late for your office, school or school. Try to understand: to lose weight, you do not need to take action that is unnatural or against your will or that you do not like. Weight loss should be integrated into your normal body processes and habits.

Wake up every morning and go to your office or university, school or workplace. This requires some practice. Contact your needs at the workplace or school. This requires a natural exercise on your part. If hours or periods are specifically allocated to exercise, when large groups of people routinely practice together, the better. Although no such hours were set aside, not at all. Remember that your body performs exercises all day when you go from home to your workplace; when you come back from work; when shopping in a supermarket; when you go to a friend; when you go to the library and return the book; when you bathe; when mowing the lawn; when using rakes and shovels in the garden and driveway; while cycling to a nearby location.

This is the beauty of natural exercise. Most things happen when you are unconscious while doing the things you normally do. Natural training does not require a strict regime and does not require you to spend money. When you feel you feel no mental or physical tension. Natural training is therefore extremely beneficial and beneficial.

Don't eat too much

Moreover, a slim figure cannot be achieved by practice alone. The most important ingredient for achieving a slim figure is diet control. If you only exercise and do not regulate your diet, you remain as fat as ever. Diet control, of course, does not mean hunger.

Do not cut meat for slicing slats

Surgery for weight loss is not recommended at all. If you are overly obese, this may be the only way out. However, an operation to remove fat layers is not desirable at all. People who try and cannot lose weight go to surgery. But the most important thing is that they can avoid surgery .

if they are trying to lose weight properly if they read this Book on how to lose weight. Surgery is an invasion of the body and can cause many complications. Doctors and surgeons have always said that surgery is the best way out for corpulent people. It is not true. Doctors and surgeons have a lot to gain by acting on you in the form of medical fees, medical fees, etc. That's probably why they will talk about the operation right away. They describe the surgical process as simple because it takes no more than 45 minutes.

Operations performed on fat people or anyone else can be quite scary. If something goes wrong, the patient can die, which can become so dangerous. And if everything goes well, you will still have to go through routine postoperative pain, trauma, and discomfort. So, before you register with a document that has been given to you by the hospital and agree to lose weight due to surgery, you need to think for a while. If you know the tricks of weight loss, you don't have to enter the operating room. If you read this book, the surgeon may not let the scalpel pass through your meat.

Spice Up Slimming by Eating Your Favorite Food

Now let's talk about food. Yes, you can use your favorite foods to lose weight. Never think of giving up pasta, chocolate, cream soup, ice cream, steaks, bacon, salami, sausages, butter, jam, cheese, mutton, biryani or any favorite meal. If you deny what you like best, you will feel robbed and sick in your mind. If you do not eat your favorite meals for days, you will feel depressed and you must contact other doctors to prevent depression. No, it's not like that. Driving and denial are not the way to go. It won't get you anywhere. If you robbed for two weeks, you will feel that you are eating the food that you refused in the next two weeks. Net result: quickly turn on the two kilograms or pounds you could spill. What You Do Eating refill every day, but your favorite meals until the weekend. Eat cereals, lentils, lean meats and fruits, and fatty foods only on weekends during the week. Pay attention to this eating discipline and you will see that it will be miracles for you!

Don't let your mind get depressed if you want your body to get depressed.In the end, you don't feel depressed. Weight loss is a breeze. Those who say it is hard to lose anything. Or they did it wrong.

There are two primary reasons why most people lose weight. One is to look good. The second is to stay healthy. Because most organs, including the heart and kidneys, break up if you're overweight. Obesity also causes diabetes, hypertension and other health problems. Those who feel depressed because they are fat fall into the category of people obsessed with their appearance. The appearance is external. I think that if your health is at risk for obesity, if the meat is a serious health risk, then this is understandable.

But be disturbed because you don't look slim and hip! It's ridiculous. Appearance is not everything! Don't get me wrong. I'm not trying to tell you how ugly you look. I try to say that: You never feel bad because you are fat. Never let hunters and jokes aimed at the stomach improve. You like food. It is well. It shows that you have a healthy appetite and therefore a healthy mind. Do not create miscellaneous that you have food. You will be asked and tell anyone who does with you: Yes, I am fat because I love to eat. I can smart and love waiting. And that is true. You can continue to eat what you like and still look slim only if you read and follow this weight loss guide.

Part 2: Weight Loss/Slimming Down: 8 Simple Steps

Before starting to lose weight, consider whether your

thyroid is normal. You may suffer from hypothyroidism, a disease that causes someone to come unusually. If you have diagnosed hypothyroidism, you do not need to read this Book. This is not relevant to you. Your thyroid medications, as prescribed by your doctor, will help you automatically reduce weight.

If you do not suffer from hypothyroidism, read this book and follow the instructions it contains to regulate your weight.

Step 1: Diet

Never eat less. Always eat the cartridge. Just don't eat too high-fat foods or foods that contain trans-fatty acids.

• Breakfast: eat croissants and toasts, but not butter. Eat fruits and drink fruit juice with or without sugar. You cannot hurt this amount of sugar unless you have diabetes. Eat a boiled egg. Do not try to have an omelet or fried eggs. You can eat two slices of bacon. You can have six pieces of sausage if it's chicken sausage, and two if it's pork. Try skipping jam and cheese. If the bread is too blunt without butter and jam, soak it in sugared tea or coffee or milk to get it. It has no cornflakes. It is useless because it does not fill the stomach. You can have porridge if you want. If you prefer Asian breakfast, you can contend with idlis and put it. Idlis and Valley are always welcome because they are virtually fat-free. But if you have an Asian breakfast, stick to the Asian breakfast. Don't try to mix Asian and European breakfasts. Eventually, you will eat too much and become chubby.

• Priority breakfast: You must have plenty of bread with tea or coffee to fill your stomach, otherwise you will be hungry right after breakfast. A boiled egg is a must. Fruit and fruit juices are important.

STEED

• Priority breakfast: You must have plenty of bread with tea or coffee to fill your stomach, otherwise you will be hungry right after breakfast. A boiled egg is a must. A few idlis and a small trough would be good. Fruit and fruit juices are important.

• Lunch: Stay on the main course. Be it steak and vegetables or fries and vegetables or some chicken preparation and vegetables. do not have thick cream soup. Always take supplies and light soups with bread or breadsticks.

Don't eat dessert. For lunch and dinner, it is always better to have Asian dishes. European food is too full of fat. Asian lunch usually consists of rice, lentil soup, vegetable preparation, chicken curry, and sour curd. At the end of the meal, you do not eat sweets or sweet yogurt.

• Lunch is preferred: rice, lentil soup, vegetable

preparation, chicken curry, and sour curd. Eat as much of this lunch as you want to avoid being hungry after eating. This lunch is almost fat-free and at the same time very nutritious and helps you lose weight.

• Tea: some tea or coffee and some soft white bread. No tea cakes, please.

• Tea is preferred: it is better to skip the tea completely. If you have a hearty lunch, such as that described in the "Priority Lunch" section, you do not need anything for tea.

• Dinner: Stay on the main course. You may have sizzler, steaks, schnitzel or fries, but none of them is desirable. You don't have to eat soup more than once a day. An Asian dinner would be best to lose weight. Let's go straight to "Preferred Dinner". If you ate rice for lunch, try to have it for dinner and vice versa.

• Dinner preferred: Roti (unleavened bread). 4-5 pieces if you are tall. 2-3 pieces if they are short. Valley or lentil soup is a must. Vegetable preparation and some chicken with 2 whole potatoes. Some cucumbers, tomatoes, broccoli, lettuce, and onions like lettuce. no cream or ham in salad. If you are still hungry, take more put and salad. But have nothing but a fixed quota of cooking roti or vegetables or chicken. no desserts. no assessment.

Important: Do not touch alcohol because the alcohol is very thick. If you like soft drinks, drink orange juice or lemonade or other fruit juice instead. You can use cold drinks to steal your desire for hard drinks, but cold drinks also thicken, though not as much as alcohol (hard drinks). And they never have "Diet" labels or cold drink versions. They cause cancer and other diseases.

The above diet was established after many consultations and based on experience. It is very good for health because it is large and nutritious. It is a perfectly balanced diet and provides the human body with all the necessary nutrients such as proteins, vitamins, minerals, iron, calcium, phosphorus, carbohydrates, energy and fat.

The human body needs a small amount of fat to survive and be resistant to infectious diseases. A fat-free diet is dangerous for the body. The diet prescribed above takes this into account. It is defined so that you can consume as little fat as is important to you. It is also approved by doctors, specialists and diabetologists. It helps you stay slim and extremely fit. A diet with a prescribed diet can continue for a long time because the prescribed diet, ie, the things listed in the "Preference" section, does not damage the heart, helping you stay lean and healthy. The prescribed diet also helps to keep triglycerides, cholesterol, and sugar low and good cholesterol low to some extent. However, this prescribed diet is not specific to people with heart problems, hypertension, and diabetes.

Step 2: Indulgence

Eat food as prescribed above on all weekdays. When Saturday and Sunday arrive, you can have ONE of your favorite meals every day. If your favorite dishes are chocolate and steaks, you can have a chocolate bar on Saturday and steaks on Sundays. If your favorite foods are ice cream and biryani, you can eat ice cream on Saturdays and biryani on Sundays.

Step 3: No crashing of the diet

NEVER Go to CRASH. Emergency food is very harmful to the organism. If you suddenly stop eating for a few days or just eat breakfast and skip lunch and dinner for several days in a row, you will have a lot of trouble. The emergency diet reduces the body's immune system and makes it susceptible to viral and bacterial infections that are contagious and airborne, such as influenza, tuberculosis, colds and coughs, and even swine flu. You can even faint from the emergency diet.

Step 4: No hard diets

Never try slimming. the effect may be fatal. 'Hard weight loss' becomes heavy on your body and exposes your body to torture as a result of long-term hunger. Keep in mind that the nutritional structure prescribed in steps 1 and 2 can be carried out for a long time because it is good for body and soul. The prescribed dietary structure helps promote health and helps reduce snails and rounded tripe. You can look slim, good and healthy and in shape. The prescribed diet is good for the heart and also helps to keep sugar levels under control. not smart smiling.

Hard weight is too hard for your body. Models have often practiced this. In severe weight loss, people starve for days and try to survive only on liquids such as tea or soups.

This can be disastrous for the body. It can cause bulimia anorexia, a terrible eating disorder that can vomit you and eventually kill you. Fluid survival for only a long time can lead to massive heart attacks and premature death. Various models and supermodels died of bulimia anorexia and heart attack after practicing weight loss to look slim.

Step 5: Do not put long holes

Never expose long golds between target hazards. You can skip the tea, but never forget to skip breakfast, lunch or dinner. All these three meals are essential. If you think you can only rest by eating two meals a day, think again. Long openings between meals and one or two main meals a day cause ulcers. Stomach ulcers are very hot and can cause severe bleeding in the stomach. And wounds can become malignant and cancerous. And cancer can cost your life. Even if the ulcer does not become malignant, the treatment you need to take to prevent your ulcer from becoming malignant can be annoying. Gastric ulcers are not recommended to give holes, eat a lot of food, drink a lot of milk. Therefore, patients suffering from peptic ulcers are often obese because no restrictions can be imposed on the diet! So it would be very good if you had stomach ulcers!

Step 6: Exercise Naturally

Natural training is recommended. See Part 1: Practice Reasonably and Normally More Information on Natural Training. As far as sport is concerned, I suggest that you do only one thing that allows natural sports.

That is the only restriction I impose. Don't take your car to the office. Use public transit instead. Traveling by public transport is very good for your health. USE LIFTING. Walking on several floors can hurt your heart. Even if your office is on the second floor, I recommend using the elevator. Many people tend to walk up or downstairs in a building and enter their office.

They think they can lose a lot in this way. However, this is not a good way to lose weight because climbing floors can even harm people's hearts without heart problems.

Therefore, keep in mind the following points when exercising:

• You do not have to get up early

• No need for yoga

• Do not drive for miles

• You don't have to run

• No need to run on the conveyor belt

• You do not need to lift weights

• No need to go to the gym

• No stairs required

• You do not need to sweat your pants

• Stop using the car. Use public transit instead.

• Do not practice training. Be natural.

Step 7: Trust your eyesight

Weight depends on height. When you surf the Internet or visit a dietitian or doctor, you can easily get "length" charts that show what a person's weight should be according to their height. While you can track these charts as you lose weight, I have to tell you that it is better to use these charts only as reference documents and not as strict codes of conduct.

After all, your eyes are the best estimator of whether you look chubby, chubby, fleshy, lameness, fleshy, voluminous, bold, obese or obese. The length table can only serve as a guide. The real determining factor is your own eyes. So if you don't think you're fat when you stand in front of a mirror, then trust yourself. Even if you are fat by the data and statistics of the "height" table. Always trust your eyes. Your own eyes, mind you.

Do not go through the eyes and opinions of others. People who don't like you might say you're fat if you're just a little chubby just to get you depressed. That is why you are the best judge in deciding whether you should reduce or not.

Step 8: Be patient

Finally, relax and take it easy. Life is a very big thing. So don't let anything less important, like fat, improve from you. Be patient when you lose weight.

COMPLETE WORKOUT PROGRAMS FOR BEGINNERS AND ADVANCED PROFESSIONALS WITH INSTRUCTIONS AND ADVICE FOR YOUR TRAINING.

There is no complete fitness program for beginners because everyone is different. However, there are a few tips that you can take into account when starting a training program so that you can adapt relatively quickly.If you decide to start a fitness program, it's good for you. Now it's time for fitness and it's never too late to start. There are a few steps you need to take to start a training program. Let's look at them.

Step 1: consult your doctor

This is very important because if you sit for a while, you don't want to do anything that will hurt you. Before you start, maintain a good physical condition to see if strenuous exercise is a contraindication.

Step 2: Start Slowly

Health is the most important reason for participating in the training program. If you have been sitting for some time, you will not train for two hours on the first day. You are just ashamed and you can even hurt yourself, so you do not have to do any exercises for a while, so you immediately scratch again. Therefore, any fitness program for beginners should be relatively simple.

But don't worry. As you continue, your body adapts quickly and you can determine the pace.

Step 3: Include the right things in your beginner's fitness program

The first time you start, you may want to start with just a walk. Even five to 10 minutes of the first day will give you a good start.

As you progress through the workout program, you add strength training exercises and also stretch, warm-up and cool down so you don't get hurt. But it's easy. First, set up simple goals like running 10 minutes each day. You can build from here. Your goal is to do at least 20 minutes of some training every day, preferably one hour.

Step 4: Always sweat

Do not enter too much intensity during exercise. Your goal should be to break a good sweat and keep it running every day for 20 to 30 minutes. You must also be able to talk to people when you exercise, but not comfortably. In other words, you have to be a little breathless when exercising.

Step 5: Switch it up

As your body gets used to certain types of exercise, it becomes more effective with them, which means that your body level will decrease if you continue to use the same type of exercise. So change your cardiovascular and strength exercises in daily exercise. For example, one day you might decide that you want to swim in cardiovascular exercise and work out weight training quads. The next day you might want to ride a bike for cardiovascular exercise and do some bench presses for your strength training. And remember; Again, maintain intensity no matter what you do.

Step 6: Eat well, drink plenty of water and sleep

No exercise program ensures that you will continue to look best and feel good if you do not eat well, drink enough water and get enough sleep. Most people should shoot well over eight hours of sleep a day. Nat. Your diet should contain a lot of lean protein, complex carbohydrates and fruits, and vegetables with good unsaturated fats. It should reduce or eliminate refined carbohydrates, unhealthy foods, etc.

If you train for less than a year and want to build muscle, you can be considered a beginner. One of the most difficult things for a beginner to be right about accumulation and bodybuilding is that your muscle-building program is fine. So check out the bodybuilding program for beginners below, stick to it, and you will soon be on the right track to build your body and move on to more challenging programs.

The good thing about starting muscle building is that you will probably see the best and fastest results in the first six to twelve months (if you have the right program). This can be a very exciting time and you will see a change in your body and yourself. Follow the program below, give it 3 months and you will see really big profits. However, the only drawback is that there is no beverage. It will be difficult, but if you are willing to work hard, you will get results.

BODYBUILDING PROGRAM FOR BEGINNERS

Below are some points to consider before you start training.

Think big, but keep it realistic:

I am not trying to say that you should not try to build huge muscles, but you must set your primary goal to a realistic level so that they are reachable and measurable. There is no point in setting a goal that is beyond reach and can also be counterproductive. Think about what you will achieve in a few months, consider your current level of fitness and strength, and set the ambitions that are realistic to achieve at this time. Also consider long-term thinking, focusing on what your result should look like. Use your short-term goals to ensure long-term success

Do not expect results at night

It is normal to see results quickly. Before commencing the evaluation of the results, however, please undertake several months of training. Many people can get to where they want to be in a few weeks, but usually, it will be harder than this.

Remember that you will shape your body over time and future results are likely to be achieved if you stick.Well, since we have your goals and way of thinking right, let's look at a specific program

As a beginner for bodybuilding and muscle development, you need to have 15 different exercises that use basic movements and involve many different muscle groups simultaneously. You will need these exercises in a system of sets and reps and mix them regularly so that your body does not get used to what you want. Exercise 3 times a week and keep it up to 3 months. The best exercises you can do at the same time on different muscle groups such as squats, bench press, and pull-ups

Warm-up your body with 10 minutes of simple aerobic exercises such as walking, cycling, running, resting, etc. before each session. Don't you sweat yet? Then your body is not ready for the more demanding exercises that you need to do to build the muscles.

Sets, repetitions and rest

Start slowly in the first month of training and keep it straight. Perform several sets of exercises with 15 to 20 repetitions per minute. Increase and increase the weight with each set. Rest only 30-40 seconds between sets. Also, be sure to increase your weight a little during each exercise.

This will prevent your muscles from training too much.

When you reach the second month, complete 3-4 sets of each exercise with 10 to 12 reps in each set. Make sure you increase the weight after each set. Start training with a little more weight than in the previous workout. You should now have approximately 60 seconds of rest between sets.

In the third month, complete 3-4 sets of 8 reps in each set. As before, make sure you add weight after each set while increasing the workout load. The rest between sets should now be 60-90 seconds.

Mix your routine

If you have trouble completing 15 exercises during training, divide them into 2 separate days. However, make sure you are changing different exercises and in what order. This means that you need more training days, but it will help if the program is too challenging to start.

Important points for training

Make sure you understand how to perform each

exercise correctly and safely. The best way to do this is a pre-trained professional training program that shows you what to do and the safest way to do it.

Stretch out after each exercise. This helps your recovery, muscle growth and flexibility.During each bodybuilding session, you must first observe what part of the body you are training. The muscles you start with are the muscles that get the most effective training, so change this regularly

Save the perfect form, each repetition. If you cannot complete the movement using the perfect form for each repetition, you are using too much weight and then drop it a bit.Hold on to him. Some people will not see results until the second or perhaps the third month of training. This is perfectly normal and should be continued.

End each exercise with 10 minutes of cardio and tighten the muscles that feel tight.Once you complete the third month, you will have a very strong foundation to work with. With a well-shaped figure, you will be strong. This not only improves your body but also improves your mental state and allows you to focus on training for even better results. Once you have reached this focus, it is time for you to adjust your program to focus on larger and longer-term goals. Remember, there is not only a perfect product or program.

You will learn what works for you, how you proceed and gain more confidence in your training

This is one of the most common questions that flood my email every day. For people who have just started a bodybuilding training program, the whole process can be an amazing experience. There are so many contradictory advice on strength training and exercise that you really don't know who or what to trust.

I understand what you are going through because I experienced the same thing when I started bodybuilding 17 years ago. People always tend to complicate things than they really are. But if you put aside all the hype and go to the basics, you will see that muscle building and shaping are not too complex.

Don't get stuck by having the perfect workout routine, the exact number of sets and reps, or the perfect eating plan, etc. Just start and do it. You can find out the details and find ways to improve as you continue.

I will learn a great training program for bodybuilding beginners that you can follow. You don't need luxury equipment. In fact, you could follow this routine with a simple home gym. But if you have the opportunity, I suggest you go to a commercial fitness center.

In addition to choosing better exercise equipment, the

commercial fitness center has a lot more energy. And this will help you motivate you to stick to your workouts and make improvements.

Start training every other day. This gives your body enough time to recover and grow muscles. Weightlifting causes less damage to the muscles and then the body responds by enlarging and strengthening the muscles to meet their requirements. Muscles do not grow during exercise; grow while you relax. After training, give your body time to regenerate and build muscle. Then you repeat the process of training and rest.

A common mistake of many bodybuilders is to think that the more they train, the better the results. This is not true because what is happening is that the muscles are split, but they never get a chance to rebuild. This is what is called "about training" in bodybuilding. If you exercise too much, your body cannot build new muscles and you can even lose part of the muscle mass you now have.

Here is a good routine with a solid workout you can follow. With this routine, you divide your workouts by training your upper body during the first workout and then training your lower body during the second workout.

WORKOUT 1: (upper body)

Bench Press 3 sets of 10 reps (chest)

Lat Pull Downs 3 sets of 10 reps (for reversal)

Arm seat press 3 sets of 10 reps (for shoulders)

Bicep Barbell Curls 3 sets of 10 reps (for biceps)

Triceps Push Downs 3 sets of 10 reps (for triceps)

WORKOUT 2: (lower body)

Leg Press 3 sets of 10 reps (for quadriceps)

Leg Curls 3 sets of 10 reps (for hamstrings)

Add 3 sets of 10 reps (for quadriceps)

Stand Calve raises 3 sets of 15 reps (for calves)

Abdominal crunches 3 sets of 25-50 reps (for abs)

With this routine, you train every other day and change two training routines. For example: perform exercise 1, take a rest day, perform exercise 2, take a rest day, and repeat the exercise with exercise 1.

Before each exercise, make 1 or 2 light heating kits with approximately half the weight you would normally use for your work kit. The weight you are lifting in the first few weeks should be low enough to easily complete the repetition. Then gradually increase the weight you are lifting.

A good goal would be to add 5 lbs. every exercise every week. For larger exercises such as bench, push-ups, press press, etc. This will be quite easy, but for smaller exercises such as biceps scrolls and triceps push-downs, it may not always be possible to use these 5lb low weight jumps. There is a big difference between adding 5 lbs. for pressing feet 250 pounds compared to adding 5 pounds. up to 25 pounds biceps curl. Remember and do everything possible to increase your strength whenever possible.

Seven-step fat burning program for beginners
The only way to burn fat and lose weight is to eat healthily and exercise. So what training program should you start if you are a complete beginner? You need to find a program that is created specifically for beginners. If you try one that is not, it can hurt your body and discourage you from trying other weight loss programs. Here is a specially designed plan for beginners that delivers amazing long-term results. It is a ninety-five-day exercise program that consists of seven parts. When you enter each part, you burn more calories and lose weight.

- You can perform any action during the first part. You can clean your house, jog or walk. Everything that moves you. You must exercise some form of physical activity for 15 to 45 minutes at a time, but only until you have reached a total of 90 minutes within the first five days of the program start. You can then proceed to the second part of the program.

- In the second part of this program, you need to deepen your physical activity. This part lasts fifteen days. For example, you have to run faster, run faster or clean the house faster. You have to practice for 30 to 60 minutes each day until you have completed a total of five hundred minutes of exercise by the end of fifteen days. You can then proceed to the third part of the program.

- During Part Three, you need to step up your activities even more. You should run instead of jogging or choosing other activities like swimming. You have to choose the things you want to do. This part lasts fifteen days. You do heavy exercise 30 to 20 minutes a day and light exercise 45 to 40 minutes a day until you reach a total of five hundred and twenty minutes of exercise at the end of fifteen days. You are now ready for Part Four.

- In part four, do two back-to-back exercises. You need to do heavy exercise for thirty to twenty-five minutes and then light forty to sixty minutes a day. You will do this until you reach a total of six hundred and seventy-five minutes after the end of fifteen days. For example, ride thirty-five minutes fast and then run slowly for twenty minutes. You can take a 15-minute break if necessary. You are now ready for the fifth part of the program.

- In the fifth part, you do two different exercises, but at different times of the day. You must spend at least three hours between the two training sessions. Perform heavy activity for 30-45 minutes.

Then carry out a lighter activity later for thirty to sixty minutes. You practice sixty to one hundred and five minutes a day. You do this every day until you reach a total of six hundred minutes of training at the end of fifteen days. You can now proceed to the part of the sixth program.

- In section six, you can only perform medium to heavy activities. It is not easy. You practice forty-five to sixty minutes each day. After fifteen days you have to train for seven hundred minutes. You are now ready for the seventh part of the program. This will be the last part of the program.

- In section seven, complete two medium and heavy exercises at different times of the day. You perform an average or strenuous activity for 30-40 minutes. Then wait at least three hours for your next workout. Then perform another exercise for thirty to twenty-five minutes until you reach a total of nine hundred minutes at the end of the fifteen days.

Always consult your doctor before starting any exercise program. As with all workouts, eat a healthy diet to burn fat and maintain weight loss. Many professional athletes regularly do weight exercises. This is because exercise on weight gain greatly improves strength, stamina, and stamina.

Many beginners assume that weight training is difficult after seeing training points with Hindu squats/handles, burpees, and cervical bridges. However, these advanced exercises are equally advanced! For beginners, a very simple exercise program can work wonders.

The results he only brings from squats, sit-ups, push-ups, and nipples can be surprising. On the other hand, the results should not be so surprising as these exercises affect almost every muscle group.

And advanced or not, if you force yourself to complete a decent circuit with these exercises, you are not wrong, you will feel it in every part of your body.

Let's take a closer look at the program and the exercises it carries.

The handles work on the entire upper body, including the arm, back, and chest. Conversely, squats work on the lower body including glutes, quad, and calves.

A simple crisis or sit-up develops the abs that make up the core of the body. Then there's a chin. Undoubtedly, chins increase the endurance and strength of the upper body to an incredible degree.

Every man wants a classic bodybuilder. However, they may not always know how to do this. Professional bodybuilders have the time and sometimes are blessed with genetics to isolate and touch any muscle by routine training that allows them to achieve their desired physique.

For most people with full-time work, families, and genetic makeup, unlike bodybuilding professionals, there is no happiness on their side and therefore need the best information they can get to reach their dream body.

The first thing you need to know about bodybuilding is that it requires patience, consistency, and a good diet. Once you understand the above, the next step is to create a training or training plan for beginners to help you achieve your goals without delving into your impatience for results. Before you start exercising, it is important to ensure that you do stretching exercises to prevent damage to your body muscles and strain your tendons when you start your tendon.

ROUTINES FOR MUSCLE BUILDING
Targeting for all muscle areas, upper and lower: arms, chest, shoulders, back, core, quadriceps, back thighs muscles, glutes and calves.

For those that are serious about trying to gain more

muscle and improve body shape and health should follow an organized training routine. Routine muscle-building exercises can best be explained as a program that accurately describes which exercises should be performed at what times, as well as the number of specific exercises and how you organize and distribute your exercises. A well-developed routine will contain clear instructions about which parts of your body you are working at specific times, as well as an accurate explanation of rest periods, eating habits, and muscle grouping. A well-developed and reliable muscle building routine is worth its weight in gold and can make the difference in your search for a better shape and a better future.

One of the most important points to keep in mind when training muscles is this - avoid too much at all costs. While this may seem like a good idea to work with your body as much as possible in the beginning, it is a very bad decision in the long run and can lead to many road problems.

By following a clear program that divides your muscle groups into different areas, you can prevent complications and injuries that can occur during exercise. Excessive use of certain parts of the body is a major mistake of many beginning muscle builders and is one of the main reasons professional practice should always be followed. It is much better to learn from the start in the right way than to make mistakes that can cost you a lot - both in the short and the long term.

A professional muscle-building routine splits your workout week with muscle group splitting on different days, often scattered with rest days for your muscles to recover. It is important to perform the right exercises for certain parts of your body because some exercises work with many different muscle areas at the same time, and it can be very easy to overdo part of your body without knowing it. A good muscle-building program will solve all these problems for you as it may take a while before you become familiar with your anatomy to know all this information yourself and include it in your muscle-building routines.

There are several amazing muscle building programs online, complete with instructions on every aspect of building muscle, losing fat and getting the desired body shape.

It is normal for men to build a muscular chest. Not all boys want to train their breasts for a variety of reasons, but the fact is that all boys want a nice breast. You know that a well-built chest or chest muscles immediately attract a considerable amount of attention, which in turn raises your heat meter to a higher level. This is because the male breast is considered to be one of the most beautiful features of a man. And with this feature thoroughly diluted and defined all girls will certainly play gaga.

Another thing to consider now is to find the best way to build chest muscles. This method must be effective and safe. You will not be treated with steroids here, so if you are looking for it you will not get anything.

There is an effective way to build chest muscles. When exercising and working on the chest, consider the chest anatomy. The chest is composed of four muscle areas, and if you do not work all of these muscle areas into your weightlifting procedures, you may not be able to build up your chest muscles so quickly. To manage each muscle group well, an effective workout plan must be followed to achieve good results.

Splitting the chest area into four less manageable areas is the key to properly building the chest muscles. These chest muscles are the upper pectoral muscle, the lower pectoral muscle, the inner pectoral muscle, and the outer pectoral muscle. Your goal is to develop these individual parts individually and one by one. This will ensure more intensive training for each of them and the results will appear faster.

So how do you build chest muscles by recognizing these four areas? Easy. Follow the simple breast training regime that addresses each muscle group. Here are some recommended exercises for chest muscle building:

Chest

To create muscles of the upper chest, your routine exercises should include an incline dumbbell bench press and a dumbbell. You can also choose a military dumbbell press to create the best effect.

Lower chest

For the lower chest muscles, the best exercises are bench press dumbbells, parallel bars, and dumbbells.

Internal Chest

Exercises that work out and strengthen the inner chest muscles include standing crossovers and flat flies on the bench.

Outer Chest

Exercise with flat benches and flat benches are the most suitable exercises to build muscles on the outer chest.Knowing the right chest building exercises is just the first step to achieving your goal. You must have the determination and motivation to perform these exercises regularly to get the results you always wanted. Whatever training it is, it is intensive and well done to harvest the harvest as soon as possible.

When building muscle through exercise, all muscle groups in the body must be equally focused on proper and proportional body growth. People want big muscles and cut out physics. This can be a reality when you exercise that targets all muscle groups and provides equal opportunities for their development during exercise. These exercises do not produce immediate results and therefore require patience and enthusiasm. In this case, routine training is required to perform their exercises in a disciplined manner. Exercise procedures for building a person's muscles are usually intense and long to increase muscle strength and improve overall body development.

Routine for building muscle for beginners
A beginner can follow the training routine for a perfect shape and does not necessarily increase the size and size of the body muscles. Exercise for all muscle groups would ensure that all muscle groups get used to muscle building exercises. The person who starts the exercise must make sure that it warms up well on all parts of the body. The warm-up session may take approx. 15 to 20 minutes. Examples of these exercises include running, hiking and jogging. These activities activate the muscles and prepare them for exercise.

Training for triceps

Double triceps dips

· The double rod is held with the palms facing each other. The body is supported by gluing to the rail.

· Slow down and bend slightly to support your back. You need to stay in this position for a while.

· Repeat the procedure.

Press the triceps

· Stand in front of the pulley and attach the bar to it.

· Attach the weighted clamp and then hold the bar with both hands from above

· Slide the tray down and slowly raise it

Extending the landscape of Barbell

· One is lying on the flat couch at the back

· The dumbbell is then held in the hand with the hands raised.

· Slowly bend your elbows to observe the movement of the arches and hold the barbell one inch above your forehead

· Return to the original position.

biceps training

Bicep curls

· Get up straight

· Hold the dumbbell with weights,

· Raise the dumbbell on your shoulders and then lower it slowly

Oblique bicep curls

· Sit on a sloping bench

· Hold the dumbbells with each hand

· Raise one of the dumbbells to the shoulder height

· Slow down

· Repeat the same for the other side.

Concentration curls with dumbbell

This exercise is one of the most popular and most effective in using dumbbells for ladies and gentlemen.

· Sitting vertically on a sofa or chair with feet apart and a bar on the right side of your right hand.

· Bend slightly so that the right elbow is easily placed on the right thigh.

Take your right forearm to rest on your right thigh

· Hold the bar in your right hand so that it faces you.

· Place your left hand on your left knee to maintain balance during exercise.

This bicep exercise is started by slowly twisting the right forearm to the shoulders. Performing concentration curls requires that you concentrate on the bicep muscles and make sure that your arm area is being worked on.

The best exercise for the shoulder muscles

Massive shoulders create an illusory body. All fixed-arm bodybuilders always get very high points in a round of symmetry. You also look bigger than you are. In this book, I will highlight the best exercises for the shoulder muscles.

Front presses

Barbell presses are an excellent way to create front deltoids. You can do this on a blacksmith or sit using a bar. If you stand without the back of the couch, the middle and upper back will increase. because these areas should support the shoulders and upper body at work. You can also use dumbbell presses that hold more tension on the deltoid side.

Parties

This exercise works on the deltoid side. The best way to do this exercise is to tilt the side branches with dumbbells. You can hold something with one hand and lift the dumbbell with the other until it is parallel to the floor. Tilting removes tension from the neck and decreases, maintaining tension in the area you want to focus on. You can also use side branches with dumbbells. If you then increase the weight, the shoulder should be slightly less parallel to the ground to always maintain tension on the parts and keep the traps out of training.

How to Build Thigh Muscles

Muscle building requires a balanced protein-rich diet and a training program that suits them best. Proteins are important components of muscle building. So you need to consume enough foods that contain protein and protein supplements. The other two important things are good training and relaxation. Resting is equally important for muscle building. This is the moment when real muscle mass is produced. Certain specific pieces of training are designed to build the thigh muscles.

Certain exercises are designed to train the thigh and leg muscles. The gyms are well equipped with all muscle-building equipment. There are also different training techniques depending on time and stamina. Join a professional training program to guide you through the process. You must conduct thorough research before embarking on a program. Do not choose a training set that puts excessive pressure on your muscles. Thighs are an important part of your body and carefully choose your exercises to avoid overworking your muscles. Train according to your stamina and slowly increase your timing. Always strive for a slow and stable process.

There are certain points for leg training that you should keep in mind when planning to build your thigh muscles. The basic exercise for building muscle mass for quadriceps and gluteal muscles is squat exercises. Combine squats and curls of legs in normal training mode. If your lower muscles of the body are weak, select weak point training with priority to achieve your goals. You have to devote to the full development of the legs, you must train both the thighs (front) and the muscles hamstring (back). Calf exercises should also be performed for full leg training.

Another important part of the muscle-building process is to give your muscles enough rest after exercise. Rest is an essential part because muscle building only takes place during this period. Your muscles should recover from injuries after exercise. Take rest on alternate training days initially. Various nutritional products help your muscles recover quickly. Almonds contain vitamin E, which helps in the recovery process for free radicals produced during exercise. Yogurt taken with fruit helps the body recover quickly.

You have to go on a protein-based diet with a lot of water consumption. Choose lean meats, fish, vegetables, eggs, and some protein supplements. Include a good amount of fat in your diet because they also speed up the muscle-building process. Include many fiber-rich and carbohydrate-rich products in your diet. Take care of your vitamin and nutritional needs. Do not take medication to build muscle quickly because they are not a healthy process and damage your body. Certain workouts are available that focus on building your thigh muscles. Follow several regular physical activities, such as running, jumping, cycling, fast walking, because they help strengthen your leg muscles.

If you feel like building muscles and building muscles, you're not alone, because that's something many men (and even a few women!) Crave for; at the same time, you probably realized that "wanting to build and build muscles" is not the same as "build muscles". Many people who want a major part will never achieve their goals in this area, and much of this reason simply don't take the time to understand the keys that take into account muscle building; Here we look at three important keys to make sure you understand extreme muscle building.

Consistency is more important than "how much": one of the big mistakes many people make when first training to build muscles is that they push overboard during the first workout, but while it is possible to feel good early (because you have felt like you're making a lot of progress at once), it usually drops you too quickly to a place where you can't keep up with the pace; As such, it's good to realize that finding a workout that you can stay in with is much more effective than pushing so hard on a handful of workouts that you will eventually run out of workout!

Knowledge goes a long way: another big mistake people make in their attempts to grow is that they are just starting to train without learning all the little things that will ultimately change their results; It may seem that you are only slowing down to achieve the goals you set yourself, but you still need to take the time to learn as much about sports as possible to make sure you get the most out of it. the workout you do.

Lifestyle is important: Make sure you are aware that "exercising" is not enough to achieve the level of muscle you want to achieve! In addition to good exercise regularly, you also need to make sure you eat well, sleep well, reduce stress and make a good lifestyle choice; these things will help you far in delivering the results you want!

Strengthen the core and leg muscles

The reason why core strength and leg strength is important to any sport, especially skating, is that most movement and balance depend on the leg muscles and core strength. When your core and leg muscles are weak, skating is very difficult. A good balance not only keeps you calm on your feet but also helps strengthen your movements. A strong core and good leg strength mean better performance in different sports.

On the way to a strong body, remember that the body needs fuel. Your diet and exercise are equally important. Make sure you have the right amount of protein needed for optimal exercise. Keep fat intake low. Under no circumstances should you give up your carbohydrates. You need complex carbohydrates. This gives you exercise while exercising. Eat whole grains, vegetables, and fruits.

The core is the center of the strength of your body, your "energy center" and the basis of all your movements. Leg muscles are equally important for maintaining balance. These are the muscles that lift your leg aside, your toes and keep you moving forward. It is important to keep these muscle groups strong.

The primary kidnapper lifting the leg to one side is the gluteus medius; This muscle is extremely important for skaters. As you strengthen the core and leg muscles, balance can improve. The muscles that make up the core, pelvis, and hips must be strong to function effectively.

You need to work on the core muscles to develop core strength. This requires you to do much more than your traditional crisis. You can perform movements such as Surface exercises where you face down on the forearm pad with the palms on the floor. As you push the floor, raise your toes and lean on your elbows. Make sure your back is flat in a straight line from head to toe. Tilt the pelvis and put the abdominal muscles together to prevent the back from sticking in the air.

Hold the position for at least 20 to 60 seconds, slow down and repeat for 3-5 reps. Exercise plank is a great way to build stamina in your stomach and back. It also helps stabilize muscles. Lie on your back with your knees bent during the bridge exercise. Keep your back in a neutral position, bent and uncompressed into the floor. Tighten the abs while lifting your hips off the floor until your hips are level with your knees and shoulders. Hold three deep breaths. Another good core exercise is the Russian move.

This is done by sitting on the floor and placing the feet under a stable surface. With your knees bent, bring your stomach back and keep your torso straight. Move your hands from one side to the other with one hand on the other and straight arms. Don't stop in the middle. Make sure you breathe well; Don't hold your breath. You can do this exercise with weight for a more intense workout. Superman exercise is good for the lower back and is a good and useful way to improve your balance.

While holding one arm and leg against the floor, fully extend the opposite arm and leg. Pull the muscles and buttocks of the back. The big advantage of good basic strength is that you don't have to worry about problems with your back or hip muscles, which can lead to other injuries. Your chances of missing an ice age are minimized. Core strength can be improved by working in the middle of the body. Basic exercises help. You strengthen your core muscles. Every exercise that uses your body without support helps. The lower body contains some of your largest muscle groups that can carry significant weight. Good balance also means strong leg muscles.

The main muscles of the lower body for good balance are your hips and quadriceps. Exercises for these muscles include hip abduction. To strengthen the front of the legs, you can perform exercises for bone pressure, straight legs, and knee lengthening.

Hip Abduction: This exercise strengthens the muscles of the outer, upper limb. This exercise is for the inner thigh. This is done in a fixed position. To do so, keep your hip straight and move the thigh in towards the centerline of the body. This exercise works like the largest hip muscle and femur.

Leg Press: Use your abs to lift your legs in an arched position directly above your head. Repeat until the required number of retries is completed. This is a useful exercise for ATVs, but it also works hamstrings and glutes.

Raising straight legs: Tighten the quadriceps muscles on the front of the thigh. Wait 10 seconds. Relax and relax for three seconds.

Knee Extensions: Sit on your chair with your back to your back. If your feet lie flat on the floor in this position, place a rolled towel under the knees and lift them. Only the balls on the feet and feet should rest on the floor. Place your hands on your thighs or hips. It takes three seconds and stretches the right leg in front of you parallel to the floor until the knee is straight.

With your right leg in this position, bend your foot so that your toes point toward your head; Keep your foot in this position for at least three seconds. Spend five seconds lowering your right leg back to the starting position so your football rests on the floor. Repeat with left leg. Change the legs until you have performed the exercise 10 to 15 times with each leg.

The squat is the best exercise for leg strength. Stand with your feet shoulder-width apart, with your toes slightly outward, with dumbbells or a dumbbell behind your neck and over your shoulders. Keep your head vertical, your back straight and your feet in full contact with the floor, bend towards your hips and move your buttocks backward until your thighs are parallel to the floor. Don't let your knees stick out in front of your toes. While maintaining that posture, bring your hips forward while returning to a standing position.

Lunge: Hold dumbbells on your shoulders, stand with your feet shoulder-width apart. Hold your head vertically and back straight before one leg forward and bend to the knee until your front leg is a 90-degree angle and the knee on your back leg almost touches the floor. Return to a vertical position and change legs. Keep the right shape again and do not let the front knee pass in front of your toes. Try to keep a long pass for better results.

Deadlift focuses on the entire back chain. The feet should be placed in the armpit width with the toes slightly outward. Skins are placed next to the line. Most of the bodyweight should start on the feet with a transfer to the heels by locking. The hands should grip the rod with an over / under grip with the arms outside the knees. The legs should be bent approx. 60 degrees from vertical with hips lower than shoulders. Your head should look forward to a neutral position.

The chest should be forward, not down. Shoulders should be pressed firmly backward and placed directly over the bar. Not around the shoulders, because then more force is exerted on the back. Stand behind the bar so it is above your feet. Keep your feet shoulder-width apart, pointing forward or slightly outward. Cover down and grab the rod, hands slightly larger than shoulder-width apart.

Thighs should be approximately parallel to the ground, straight back and eyes forward. Keep your back rigid and your arms straight, lift the bar with your legs and hold the bar as close as possible to your body.

Balanced exercises help to maintain strong core and leg muscles and prevent falls. The leg consists of several parts. Quadriceps are the muscle group on the front of the thigh above the knee used to extend the knee, hamstrings are a group of muscles on the back of the thigh, doing the opposite and bending or pulling the knee.

Calves are a group of muscles located on the lower limb along the back of the tibia. They are used to extend the ankle or to lift the heel while standing. All leg muscles work together to create speed and movement. They work in a combination of strength, acceleration, and speed. Every muscle is important. Not only do you train a muscle group, do them all. Strong leg muscles, especially for quadrilaterals, hamstrings, and calves, are important for figure skating. Most of your strength comes from your legs and you also need strong leg muscles to maintain balance.

If you want to increase your core and leg strength for better balance, your quads, hamstrings, and abs are the muscles to focus on. Exercises such as Russian pull and sit and crunch are good. The Plank helps to strengthen the core; Try holding it for about 30 seconds at a time and increase as you become stronger. Things like lifting feet also help. Remember, it is important to maintain a high-protein and low-fat diet in any routine workload to improve muscle growth and development, otherwise, you will not get anywhere. Focus on overall fitness and maintaining a healthy regime.

Healthy eating does not beat anything. Eat a combination of lean proteins and complex carbohydrates. Expand your food. Your metabolism is a machine that works constantly. He needs fuel. Eat smaller meals every few hours during the day to speed up fat loss and maintain a steady energy level. For best results, eat six smaller meals a day. Eat your proteins, lean chicken, fish, proteins and beans. You have to consume so many fruits and vegetables. Drink at least three liters of water a day. Soda is your worst enemy, diet or not. During the repetition, focus on the overall strength of the body with an emphasis on core and leg strength.

However, I will spend some time reviewing the best practices that you can implement and help you in your quest for muscle mass. This will help you achieve remarkable results and you may be one of the few people who have done a good body transformation.

Lift heavyweights

If you want some great muscle building tips, I suggest you listen carefully. This is valuable information about building muscle mass. Yes, you've probably heard it before, you need to lift heavy weights to gain muscle. However, not only does heavyweight help, but also the exercises you choose. If you want to be sure that you build as many muscles as possible, you must involve deadlift and squat in the exercise.

If you are looking for one or two exercises that are best for building muscle throughout your body, then it's a squat and deadlift. I know you could think, but don't you focus primarily on your feet? The answer is a little yes and a little no. Imagine you are doing a squat. Do you see that all the weight you have at the bar lifts your entire body? Yes, you are right, your squat is using your entire body. True, your legs are the main goal of shifting this weight, but your other muscles must support your body to do a squat.

Another reason is that squat and deadlift are one of the few exercises where you can lift a huge amount of weight. Because these exercises work throughout your body and you can use a lot of weight, it causes a huge release of growth hormones that make your body grow. These are the reasons why doing squats and deadlifts will help increase muscle mass throughout the body.

Avoid injury

As we have already mentioned, lifting is essential for

muscle mass growth. However, you also need to be careful to continue training that is too long without taking a break. If you do this for too long without a break, you can topple you.

As you may already know, muscle exercise can cause muscle loss or deterioration. There's nothing worse than when you want to train, but it's not possible because of injury. This usually means that your muscle gains are stopped and you have to concentrate on healing injuries. This may cause you to stop training for a while. You can imagine how many potential muscles were lost after this amount of free time.

What you need to do is spend a week so often that it is easy to exercise. During the week of stretching, foam rolling and perhaps a few light exercises pay attention.

Change your exercise program

This tip is more or less related to the things I mentioned earlier. But I felt it fit into his part as well. What this tip is about is training exercises and body parts that you like and positioning them last, and placing the exercises and body parts you will encounter at the beginning of the exercise. Why is this important? People often have weaknesses, and when you first train your strong areas, they become stronger and your weak areas become weaker. This can help you focus on your weaknesses when you have full energy, so you can give all the exercises in which you are the weakest. Over time, your weak areas can turn into strong areas.

If you want to build muscle quickly, we strongly recommend that you apply these tips in practice. By concentrating on gradual overload, pumping heavy iron, using it for weeks to prevent injury, and inflating your workout program to make your body strong, you're on your way to your amazing body transformation.

3 WEEKS OF WEIGHT LOSS TRAINING TO GET FAST FAT BURNING AND STRENGTH RESULTS.

Here's a 3 weeks workout program to help you burn fat and gain muscle. You will do fat burning exercises in short workouts to get maximum results in minimal time.

You need to take the time to plan and prepare your fitness and weight loss diet and exercise program for the rest of the week. But if you haven't already, here's a 7-day workout to help you burn fat.

You must also head to the supermarket to shop and prepare food for the next 3 weeks and plan your next 3 weeks of fitness by following these instructions.

Monday

Do fitness training for strength and range.

Warm-up your body weight to get started.

Then replace one-leg exercises such as split squats and dumbbells. Perform 3 sets of 8.

Afterward superset stability ball bone curls with rows of the dumbbell. Makes 3 sets of 12.

Stop the interval cardio workout. Fat burning takes only 20 minutes.

Tuesday

Get 30 minutes of fun exercises. It can be traditional cardio, shopping, housework, crafts or your favorite sport. Make sure you are active every day. Stop your activity with some relaxation techniques. It can be a deep breathing, some simple yoga poses or some visualization methods. Whatever you do, take a few minutes to relax and relax the stress of your day.

Wednesday

Perform the next exercise at strength and intervals - very similar to Monday training. Combine your workout between two protein-rich snacks to get the muscles the nutrients they need to regenerate and replenish.

Thursday

30 minutes of activity. Check the vegetable intake. You should get at least 5 servings a day, but try to get up to 8 or even 10 servings a day. Focus on green wheatgrass.

Friday

Your last workout of the week.

Weight training is hot right now and is quickly becoming a (busy) people choice as a training method to help them get the slim, slim and sexy figure they always wanted. Besides, you will probably want to spend less time at the gym and more time outdoors at this time of year.

So today, do only exercise with body weight.Start with a superset of Bulgarian split squats and chin-ups. The second superset can be handles and front lungs. If you want, do a few biceps and triceps exercises for fun.Thereafter the interval cardio is performed for 20 minutes.

Saturday

30 minutes of activity. Connect with your social support group. And call another friend and encourage them to commit to losing fat and improving their health. Help them and compare obstacles that prevent you from eating or exercising.

Sunday

30 minutes of activity followed by a weekly program, storage, and preparation. Check your diet and make sure all sources of trans fats from your diet. Get rid of all light foods that contain trans fat and other ingredients you can't pronounce. Focus on fresh products and minimize pre-packed foods on your list.Repeat this for the 3 weeks to get Fast Fat Burning and Strength results.

CONCLUSION

Calisthenics is a form of training where people use only their body weight to gain strength and be fit. Calisthenics exercises can be practiced without many machines or extensive gymnastic structures. The basic idea is to gain endurance, endurance, flexibility, and power without relying on tools or advanced equipment.

Calisthenics training is designed for everyone differently based on their fitness and medical history. Undoubtedly, it is one of the most suitable fitness industries for those who have healthy health. It is this representation of muscle strength and body control that has made it a sport that many people like to practice and compete with.

Calisthenics is a versatile genre of exercise where body weight is used as resistance. The use of the machine is minimized with basic tools such as pickup and dip rods, which can be purchased locally or welded at home. Most people are attracted because these exercises can be performed almost anywhere. You can have any number of columns in the backyard and you're ready to go.

Who can practice Calisthenics exercises

Calisthenics is for everyone, but because the form is based on body strength and stamina, it needs a little training before it gets used to it. People who begin to practice and exercise may need up to six months to perform all the basic movements smoothly.

Calisthenic training can be used to achieve all kinds of health goals. Some athletes and bodybuilders train them to increase the strength and flexibility of the body. Training has different levels and can, therefore, be used to achieve all kinds of goals.

It is an ideal exercise for weight loss, muscle building, core strength, and overall coordination and body shape. Even if you do not have clear health goals and generally enjoy good health, gymnastic exercises are enough.

Calisthenics cannot be defined in one category as it includes everything that supports weight training. However, certain types of exercises can be performed at the beginner level. Once a person can do this, they can be included in circuit training or other forms to get better results.

A few examples of Calisthenics training:

Boards: Planking helps your core and abs gain strength.

Lie on the floor in the exposed position and support your weight on your feet and forearms.

Keep your body straight at all times and hold this position as long as possible. You can raise your arm or leg to increase severity.

Dips: Dips are compound exercises of weight gain. They can do wonders for the strength of your upper body, exercising your chest, shoulder, back and arm muscles.To do Dips, first, raise yourself to two dips with straight arms. Lower your body when your shoulders are below your elbows. Push in until your arms are straight again.

Squats: These are usually beneficial to the legs and mainly train the muscles of the thighs, hips, and buttocks.Stand with feet slightly wider than shoulders, hips stacked above knees and knees above ankles.

Keep your head forward with your eyes straight forward

for a neutral spine. While your buttocks protrude, make sure your back stays straight and your chest and shoulders stay upright.

Pull out: Extraction is an upper-body pull exercise. Hooks and other types will help you build your back, arms, shoulders and strengthen your core.

Grab the handle with the palms facing forwards or backward. With straight arms, separate the shoulder width. Pull up your elbows by pulling your elbows on the floor.Continue to move until the chin passes beam. Fold-down completely until your arms reach out, then pull out again.

Handle Note: For a wide grip, your hands should be more distant than the shoulder width. For average grip, the hands should be at a distance equal to the width of the shoulders and for a firm grip at a distance less than the width of the shoulder.

Push-up exercise: Push-up exercise is a common exercise for gymnastics in a stomach position by lifting the body with your hands up and down. The handles are used to develop chest and tricep muscles.

Stand on a high board position. Place your hands firmly on the floor, straight back to keep the entire body neutral.Lower the body and push upwards.

When you return to the starting position, keep your core busy, exhale.

Burpees / Squat Thrust

Burpees are all-body exercises that train practically many muscles in the body, from abs, glutes and hip flexors to the chest and shoulders. You can burn more calories in a much shorter time.

The starting position is vertical with the width of the legs apart and the hands-on sides. Sit on your knees and place your hands on the floor in front of your feet. Jump your legs in a row until they are fully extended, push all the way up once and jump your legs directly by your hands. Use an explosive motion to push the heels and return to the home position.

Explosive jumping lunges

Focus on primary muscle groups: quads and hamstrings. Secondary: abdominal muscles, calves, glutes, and hip flexors.

Stand straight with the solid core and chest up. Drop your right foot forward, place your hands on your hips and jump, move your foot in the air and land your left foot forward.

Calf lifts

Standing calf exercises focus on your calf muscles, especially the larger, outer muscle responsible for the shape and size of the calves. The calf muscles are seen as something else as an aesthetic priority.

Stand up with a solid core and a flat back.Hold your hands along your body or hold the wall for balance.

Divide your legs to the distance between your hips. Lift the heels by stretching the ankles as high as possible and bending the calf. Pause the top and slowly return to the starting position.

Hanging feet up

Foot hanging is a basic workout that focuses on the entire abdomen and improves lower-back stability and helps strengthen other muscle groups such as your arms, shoulders and even your legs.Grab the handle with a firm handle. Raise the legs so that the torso makes an angle of 90 degrees, lower the legs slowly until they are straight and repeat.

Ab Workout: Exercising abdominal muscles will help you gain more control over body movements, in addition to the attractive six-pack abs.

There are various benefits associated with AB exercises. For example, it helps the body achieve a better posture because your muscles are stronger. These exercises will also alleviate back pain and find that your lower back will be more flexible and your digestion will be improved by regular abdominal exercises.

If you are starting with a training routine to reduce excess fat, it is important to focus first on the lower abdomen, as this area is most difficult to strengthen and strengthen. The upper abs are more natural and firmer, while the lower abs are stronger.

Calisthenics is a safe and result-oriented form that works.